Herbal Teas and Natural Remedies

A Guide to Healing through the Harnessed Power of Natural Herbs

Dr. Amalie Kleist

1

Table of Contents

DISCLAIMER

This content is not meant to offer medical advice or replace advice or treatment from a personal physician. It is recommended that you get advice from your doctors or trained health specialists for any specific health inquiries you may have. Readers or followers of this instructional resource are responsible for any potential health effects.

Introduction

In a world where contemporary medicine rules the healthcare discourse, "Herbal Teas and Natural Remedies: A Guide to Healing through the Harnessed Power of Natural Herbs" with DIY recipe tips by Dr. Amalie Kleist quietly ushers in a return to our ancestors' knowledge and practices.

Dr. Kleist reveals a wealth of herbal remedies, each as distinctive as the plant it comes from, ranging from the calming embrace of chamomile to the energizing zest of peppermint. She carefully crafts recipes for tinctures, teas, and salves, enabling people to use nature's healing powers for themselves.

This book serves as a reminder of our symbiotic relationship with the natural world and a monument to the interdependence of all living things, rather than just a collection of recipes. Readers learn from Dr. Kleist's instruction that true healing is a mental, bodily, and spiritual symphony of wholeness that transcends the physical world.

With each page turn, Dr. Kleist transmits not only knowledge but also a sense of reverence for the earth's riches. She reminds us that the plants in our gardens and woodlands are more than just commodities to be exploited; they are sacred allies in our quest for health and well-being.

"Herbal Teas and Natural Remedies" is a calm haven for readers to take a break, relax, and re-establish a connection with the natural rhythms in a world of haste and strife. It exemplifies the enduring power of old knowledge and serves as a beacon of hope for all who seek healing in Mother Earth's embrace.

Herbalism, in the hands of Dr. Amalie Kleist, becomes a way of life—a philosophy based on reverence, appreciation, and great regard for the intricate web of life that nourishes us all. One sip of tea and one cure at a time, this beautiful book gives us the strength to start a journey of self-discovery and healing.

Chapter One

Introduction to Herbal Teas and Natural Remedies

Herbal teas and natural remedies have been highly valued for ages in various cultures around the world due to their therapeutic characteristics and comprehensive approach to promoting health and well-being. These remedies, derived from a variety of plants, herbs, roots, and flowers, provide a mild yet powerful alternative to traditional medicine for treating common diseases and enhancing overall health.

Herbal teas, or tisanes, are infusions created by steeping dried leaves, flowers, fruits, seeds, or roots from different plants. They are created by immersing the plant material in hot water, enabling the extraction of its advantageous components into the liquid. Herbal teas are well-regarded for their pleasant taste and wide array of health benefits. Herbal teas provide a variety of options to suit different preferences and requirements, ranging from soothing chamomile to energizing peppermint.

Natural remedies refer to a diverse range of herbal preparations, extracts, oils, and salves that are utilized to target specific health issues. These remedies utilize the therapeutic characteristics of plants to facilitate the healing process, mitigate symptoms, and bolster the body's innate capabilities. Natural medicines offer gentle and efficient solutions for common problems, such as soothing aloe vera gel for sunburns and scented eucalyptus oil for congestion alleviation.

Advantages of Natural Remedies and Herbal Teas

Holistic Healing: Natural remedies and herbal teas handle health from a holistic perspective, addressing not only physical ailments but also mental and spiritual wellbeing.

Minimal Side Effects: Herbal teas and treatments frequently have fewer side effects than pharmaceutical medicine, which makes them a good choice for people looking for gentler options.

Versatility: Because of the large variety of herbs and plants that can be used, herbal teas and treatments are highly adaptable and can be used to treat a wide range of health problems, from skin conditions to digestive problems and stress.

Accessible and Economical: A wide spectrum of

individuals can benefit from herbal teas and natural remedies because they are frequently more easily obtained and reasonably priced than prescription drugs.

Natural Remedies

Herbal supplements: These are products made from plants, such as powders, capsules, or extracts, which contain concentrated amounts of active ingredients thought to have therapeutic benefits.

Essential Oils: Made from plants, these intensely concentrated oils can be applied physically or inhaled for a variety of uses, such as aromatherapy, skincare, and relaxation.

Homeopathic Remedies: Homeopathic remedies, which are based on the idea that "like cures like," use extremely diluted chemicals to encourage the body's natural healing mechanisms.

Nutritional Supplements: This category includes vitamins, minerals, and other dietary supplements, often used to address specific deficiencies or to support overall health.

Traditional Medical Practices: Ayurveda and Traditional Chinese Medicine (TCM), two of the many cultures that practice traditional medicine, combine natural therapies, including herbs, acupuncture, and meditation.

Herbal Teas

Camellia sinensis Teas: green tea, black tea, white tea, and oolong tea are all made from the same plant but processed differently. Each type offers unique flavors and potential health benefits due to their antioxidant content.

Herbal Infusions: They are traditionally valued for their relaxing, digestive, or immune-boosting qualities. Herbal infusions are made without caffeine from dried herbs, flowers, fruits, or spices. Teas flavored with chamomile, peppermint, ginger, and hibiscus are typical examples.

Decaffeinated Teas: Some teas are decaffeinated to remove the majority of the caffeine content, making them appropriate for caffeine-sensitive individuals.

Blended Teas: These are blends of various teas, herbs, or spices that are frequently created to achieve specific flavor profiles or health benefits. Blends for detoxification, relaxation, and immune system stimulation are a few examples.

Potential Benefits

Holistic Approach: A lot of herbal teas and natural remedies are highly regarded for their holistic approach to health, which addresses the body's fundamental imbalances as well as symptoms.

Less Side Effects: Natural remedies and herbal teas

frequently have fewer side effects than pharmaceutical medications, which makes them appealing to people looking for more gentle methods of managing their health.

Antioxidants: Herbal teas and some natural medicines are rich in antioxidants. They help fight oxidative stress and inflammation in the body and may lower the risk of chronic diseases.

Boosting Digestive Health: A number of herbs, including chamomile, peppermint, and ginger, are well-known for their ability to improve digestion, lessen bloating and gas, and calm upset stomachs.

Stress Reduction: Calming herbs like chamomile, lavender, and lemon balm are found in many herbal teas and can aid in lowering tension and encouraging relaxation.

Immune Support: It is thought that herbal teas and

supplements with components like astragalus, elderberry, and echinacea would boost immunity and help ward against or treat colds and the flu.

Better Sleep: Herbs that are frequently used to encourage relaxation and enhance the quality of sleep, such as valerian root, chamomile, and passionflower, can be helpful for people who are experiencing insomnia or other sleep disorders.

Potential Risks

Quality Control: The absence of established manufacturing techniques in herbal teas and natural treatments can result in differences in their potency, purity, and quality.

Drug interactions: Certain supplements and herbs may interact with certain drugs, reducing their effectiveness or increasing the possibility of negative side effects. It's imperative to speak with a healthcare provider before combining prescription medications and herbal therapies.

Allergic Reactions: Those who are allergic to certain herbs or plants or sensitive to them may get adverse reactions when taking herbal medicines or teas.

Toxicity: Some herbs contain substances that, when taken in large quantities or over an extended period of time, may be harmful. Examples are ephedra, which contains ephedrine, and comfrey, which has pyrrolizidine alkaloids.

Pregnancy and Breastfeeding: Because of their propensity to induce uterine contractions or transfer into breast milk, several herbs should not be used during pregnancy or nursing. When utilizing herbal treatments, people who are pregnant or nursing should use caution and speak with a healthcare professional beforehand.

Digestive Stress: Although many herbs are good for

digestion, some people who drink particular herbal teas or supplements may have negative side effects like diarrhea, nausea, or heartburn.

Herb-Drug Interactions: Some plants have the ability to alter the metabolism or effects of certain drugs. For instance, St. John's Wort may lessen the efficiency of antidepressants and birth control tablets.

When taken properly and under the supervision of medical specialists, natural remedies and herbal teas can provide significant health benefits. But it's crucial to exercise caution and balance the potential advantages against the hazards, particularly if you already have a medical problem or are taking prescriptions in addition to herbal therapies. To ensure safe and efficient use, speaking with a healthcare professional skilled in herbal medicine can be beneficial.

How to safely utilize herbal teas and natural remedies

When using herbal teas and natural medicines, there are a few important things to keep in mind. The following advice can help you minimize hazards by including these products in your wellness routine:

1. Education and research:

- *Learn about herbs:* Get knowledgeable about the herbs and components of any teas or natural medicines you are thinking about consuming. Recognize their possible advantages, drawbacks, and interactions.

- *Quality matters:* Purchase products from reliable vendors who employ standardized production procedures and place a high priority on quality control.

2. Speak with medical specialists:

- *Advice from Qualified Healthcare Professionals:* Seek advice from a qualified healthcare professional, such as a pharmacist, herbalist, or naturopathic doctor, particularly if you are taking medication, have underlying medical issues, or are pregnant or nursing.

- *Notify Your Healthcare Provider:* Since herbal teas, supplements, and natural remedies can worsen some medical conditions or interfere with pharmaceuticals, be sure to let your healthcare provider know about all of the remedies, teas, and supplements you are using or thinking about using.

3. Begin slowly and monitor:

- *Start with small doses:* To determine how your body will respond to a new tea or herbal treatment, start with a small dose. As necessary, gradually raise the dosage while adhering to the suggested guidelines.

- *Track Your Body's Reaction:* Observe how your body reacts to the teas or natural cures. Stop using the product and seek medical advice if you encounter any negative effects.

4. Pay attention to interactions:

- *Check for Interactions:* Find out if there are any possible interactions between the prescriptions you are currently taking and herbal therapies. When utilizing many herbal products at once, use caution since they could interfere with one another or prescription drugs

- *Seek Professional Advice:* Seek advice from a pharmacist or healthcare provider if you have questions regarding possible interactions.

5. Take individual sensitivities into account:

- *Allergies and Sensitivities:* Be mindful of any dietary restrictions or allergies you may have in relation to particular herbs or substances. If you have any adverse symptoms, including itching, swelling, or trouble breathing, stop using the product.

6. Follow the dosage instructions:

- *Adhere to Recommended Dosages:* Pay attention to the dose recommendations made by medical specialists or on product labels. Don't take more medication than is advised, as this may lead to more side effects.

7. Keep an eye on quality and consistency:

- *Verify Expiration Dates:* To preserve effectiveness and safety, be sure the herbal teas and natural remedies you consume are within their expiration dates.

- *Seek for Quality Certifications:* Select goods bearing approved quality certifications or that have undergone quality, purity, and safety testing conducted by respectable institutions.

8. Exercise Caution While Breastfeeding and Pregnancy:

- *Speak with a Healthcare Professional:* Before using herbal treatments or teas, anybody who is pregnant or nursing should speak with a healthcare professional because some herbs may not be safe during these times.

9. Proper storage:

- *Comply with storage Instructions:* To preserve freshness and potency, store herbal remedies and teas in accordance with the manufacturer's recommendations. Keep them out of the extremes of temperature, moisture, and direct sunlight.

10. Pay attention to your body:

- *Trust your instincts:* If anything doesn't seem right or if you get strange symptoms, follow your gut and consult a medical practitioner.

You can safely and successfully incorporate herbal teas and natural remedies into your wellness routine by adhering to these rules and taking an assertive approach. Recall that receiving individualized advice from medical specialists is crucial to guaranteeing the best possible results for your health.

Chapter Two

Herbal Teas: Types and Benefits

Herbal teas, often called herbal infusions, are brewed from dried herbs, flowers, fruits, spices, and other plant-based ingredients. They have a range of tastes and, perhaps, health advantages. The following is a list of popular herbal tea varieties and their related health benefits:

Chamomile Tea

Chamomile is well-known for its relaxing qualities, which make it a popular option for encouraging rest and improved sleep. It might also help calm troubled stomachs and facilitate digestion.

Ginger Tea

Ginger tea is well-regarded for both its potential digestive benefits and its comforting, spicy flavor. It might ease motion sickness, nausea, and indigestion. Additionally, ginger tea contains anti-inflammatory qualities.

Peppermint Tea

People frequently drink peppermint tea for its cooling taste and digestive advantages. It might ease indigestion, gas, and bloating. It may also help clear nasal congestion and headaches.

Rooibos Tea

Packed with antioxidants and naturally caffeine-free. Due

to its anti-inflammatory qualities, it may help blood sugar regulation, support heart health, and encourage good skin.

Lemon Balm Tea

This tea is well-known for its relaxing properties and has a subtle citrus flavor. It could help to reduce tension and anxiety while encouraging calm. Tea made with lemon balm may also help with digestion and enhance mental clarity.

Hibiscus Tea

This bright, crimson tea has a tangy and refreshing flavor. Because of its strong antioxidant content, it may help lower blood pressure, improve cholesterol levels, and promote liver function.

Lavender Tea

Lavender tea is valued for its soothing properties and flowery scent. It could help to reduce tension and anxiety while encouraging calm. Lavender tea can also improve your sleep quality.

Echinacea Tea

Echinacea tea is frequently drunk to boost immunity and lessen the severity and duration of colds and flu. It might also possess antioxidant and anti-inflammatory qualities.

Valerian Root Tea

Valerian root tea is well-known for its sedative properties, which can enhance sleep, lessen anxiety, and encourage relaxation. It is frequently used as an all-natural sleep aid.

Licorice Root Tea

This tea has a sweet and earthy taste. It might aid with cough relief, sore throat relief, and digestive health. However, because it may raise blood pressure, it should only be used in small amounts.

Dandelion Root Tea

It is thought to promote liver function and facilitate digestion. It might have a diuretic effect, assisting the body in getting rid of toxins. Antioxidants are also abundant in dandelion root tea.

Green Tea

Caffeine-free forms of traditional green tea can be found

in blends prepared with herbs like mint or lemongrass. They have several health advantages, such as digestive assistance and antioxidant qualities.

Cinnamon Tea

It has a warm, spicy flavor and is packed with antioxidants. It might enhance heart health, assist digestion, and help control blood sugar levels.

Passionflower Tea

Well-known for its relaxing properties, passionflower tea may aid in lowering anxiety, enhancing the quality of sleep, and encouraging relaxation. It's frequently used as an all-natural sleep aid.

Rosehip Tea

Rich in antioxidants and vitamin C, rosehip tea supports healthy skin and immune systems. It might also promote joint health and lessen inflammation.

These are only a few examples of herbal teas and the advantages they offer. Including a range of herbal teas in your daily routine can enhance your general health in addition to offering delicious flavors.

Chapter Three

Natural Remedies: Types and Benefits

A wide range of treatments made from plants, minerals, and other natural materials are included in the category of natural remedies. They are frequently used to treat a variety of medical issues and promote well-being. The following is a list of natural remedies and some of their potential benefits.

Essential Oils

Lavender Oil: It is highly valued for its ability to calm and soothe. It can ease headaches, encourage relaxation, lessen tension and anxiety, enhance the quality of sleep, and relieve skin irritations like burns and bug bites.

Peppermint Oil: It has a revitalizing and pleasant aroma.

When applied topically or aromatically, it can help ease headaches, reduce nausea, enhance digestion, ease pain and tension in the muscles, and remove congestion.

Tea Tree Oil: Tea tree oil is widely recognized for having antibacterial and antiseptic qualities. It can aid in the treatment of dandruff, fungal infections, acne, small wounds and scrapes. Tea tree oil is also used as a natural insect repellent.

Eucalyptus Oil: Eucalyptus oil smells energizing and fresh. It can relieve aching muscles, treat respiratory conditions such as colds and coughs, reduce congestion, and encourage attention and mental clarity.

Lemon Oil: It smells cheery and lively. It has the potential to elevate mood, increase vitality, sharpen focus and mental clarity, aid with digestion, and encourage detoxification.

Rosemary Oil: The perfume of rosemary oil is energizing

and herbaceous. It can aid in promoting hair development and scalp health, relieving muscle pain and tension, increasing circulation, and enhancing memory and cognitive performance.

Chamomile Oil: Chamomile oil is well-known for its relaxing and comforting qualities. It can ease skin irritations, ease intestinal discomfort, encourage relaxation and better sleep, and lessen stress and anxiety.

Frankincense Oil: Its perfume is pleasant. It is frequently used for its immune-boosting, relaxation-inducing, stress- and anxiety-relieving, calming, and grounding properties, as well as skin health benefits.

Ylang Ylang Oil: This oil has a pleasant, flowery smell. It can support healthy skin and hair, lessen stress and anxiety, encourage relaxation, lift one's spirits, and increase libido.

Bergamot Oil: Bergamot oil smells fresh and energizing. It can enhance digestion, ease skin irritations, elevate mood, reduce stress and anxiety, and encourage relaxation.

Sandalwood Oil: Sandalwood oil smells strongly of wood. It can assist emotional well-being, encourage relaxation, lessen stress and anxiety, increase mental clarity and focus, and enhance skin health.

Geranium Oil: The aroma of geranium oil is flowery and uplifting. Insect repellent, hormone balancing, mood enhancement, stress and anxiety reduction, and skin health promotion are just a few benefits.

Clary Sage Oil: The scent of clary sage oil is herbaceous and pleasant. Hormone balancing, menstrual pain relief, anxiety and stress reduction, relaxation, and healthy digestion are just a few of the benefits it can offer.

Lemongrass Oil: The aroma of lemongrass oil is fresh

and lively. It can stimulate digestion, ease tension and soreness in the muscles, repel insects, elevate mood, and enhance mental clarity and focus.

Patchouli Oil: The flavor of patchouli oil is earthy and deep. Insect repellent, mood enhancement, stress and anxiety reduction, relaxation, and skin health support are some of its benefits.

Herbal Supplements

Echinacea: It is thought to boost immunity, preventing and lessening the severity of colds and flu. It may also boost overall immunological function and have anti-inflammatory properties.

Ginseng: It is known for its adaptogenic qualities, which may help the body manage stress and encourage vigor and energy. It is also thought to enhance general wellbeing, immunological health, and cognitive function.

St. John's Wort: This herb is frequently used as a home treatment for anxiety and mild to moderate depression. It might lessen depressive symptoms, elevate mood, and support emotional health.

Ginkgo Biloba: Ginkgo biloba has long been associated with potential cognitive advantages, such as enhanced mental clarity, focus, and memory. It might also help with circulation, eyesight, and mental wellness in general.

Turmeric: The molecule curcumin, the main ingredient in turmeric, has strong anti-inflammatory and antioxidant effects. It might promote joint health, lessen discomfort, lessen inflammation, and guard against long-term illnesses.

Milk Thistle: This plant is frequently used to assist liver function and encourage the detoxification process. It might enhance liver function, shield the liver from harm, and promote general digestive health.

Valerian Root: It is a well-liked natural treatment for insomnia and other sleep disorders because of its sedative and soothing properties. It might support relaxation and enhance the quality of sleep.

Saw Palmetto: It is a popular herb used to treat benign prostatic hyperplasia (BPH) and promote prostate health. It might enhance urine flow, lessen the frequency of urination, and promote men's urinary tract health in general.

Garlic: It is known for strengthening the immune system, garlic may also promote cardiovascular health. It might improve general heart health by lowering blood pressure, cholesterol, and other cardiac-related issues.

Cranberry: Cranberry supplements are frequently used to promote urinary tract health and protect against UTIs. They may reduce the risk of UTIs by preventing bacteria from adhering to the urinary system's lining.

Black cohosh: It is frequently used as a home medicine for mood swings, hot flashes, and nocturnal sweats associated with menopause. It might aid in symptom relief and promote women's hormonal equilibrium.

Rhodiola rosea: This adaptogenic herb is thought to support resilience and energy levels while assisting the body in adjusting to stress. It might enhance general wellbeing, lessen fatigue, and enhance cognitive performance.

Holy Basil (Tulsi): Holy basil, also known as tulsi, is appreciated for its adaptogenic and stress-relieving properties. It might boost immunity, ease tension, encourage relaxation, and increase vitality.

Astragalus: It is used in traditional Chinese medicine to improve general vitality and immune function. It might strengthen cardiovascular health, lower inflammation, and strengthen the immune system.

Ashwagandha: It is an adaptogenic plant that helps the body deal with stress and promotes vigor and energy. It might support cognitive function, lessen stress, elevate mood, and increase general wellbeing.

Homeopathic Remedies

Arnica montana: Arnica is frequently used to alleviate inflammation brought on by injuries, bruises, and stiff muscles. Additionally, it might aid in reducing discomfort, swelling and hastening healing.

Belladonna: It is used to treat acute diseases that have inflammation, an abrupt start, and strong symptoms. It might assist in easing symptoms including headaches, sore throats, fevers, and earaches.

Nux vomica: Constipation, bloating, indigestion, and nausea are among the digestive problems that Nux Vomica is frequently used to treat. Furthermore, it may alleviate the symptoms caused by overindulging in food, drinks, or stimulants.

Chamomilla: It is frequently used to relieve infants' and young children's restlessness, irritation, and discomfort associated with teething. In adults, it might also ease jitters, lessen anxiety, and encourage relaxation.

Ignatia amara: It is used to treat psychological and emotional problems, including anxiety, depression, and mood swings. It might support resilience and emotional recovery in stressful or grieving situations.

Pulsatilla: It is widely used to treat respiratory infections, which include sinusitis, colds, and coughs. These illnesses typically have erratic symptoms, including thick, yellowish discharge and nasal congestion.

Hypericum perforatum: This herb is frequently used to relieve nerve pain, particularly radiating, acute, or shooting pain. It might aid in the relief of shingles, neuralgia, sciatica, and injury-related pain.

Aconitum napellus: It is used to treat acute illnesses like panic attacks, colds, fevers with abrupt onset, and flu. It might lessen symptoms including anxiety, restlessness, fever, and chills.

Bryonia alba: It is frequently used to treat inflammatory diseases that become worse with movement and get better with rest, such as migraines, arthritis, and muscle soreness. It might also help with constipation and dry coughs.

Rhus toxicodendron: It is used to treat ailments involving inflammation, pain, and stiffness in the joints and muscles. It might lessen the discomfort brought on by sprains, strains, arthritis, and restless legs syndrome.

Lycopodium: This medication is used to treat digestive problems, especially those that intensify in the late afternoon or evening, such as gas, indigestion, bloating, and constipation.

Chapter Four

Uses of Herbal Teas and Natural Remedies

There are numerous uses and advantages for herbal teas and natural remedies for general health and wellbeing.

Common Ailments and Conditions

COGNITIVE PERFORMANCE: Herbal teas with ingredients including gotu kola, ginkgo biloba, bacopa, and rosemary may assist with retention, concentration, and cognitive performance. Natural treatments for brain health and cognitive function include phosphatidylserine, acetyl-L-carnitine, and omega-3 fatty acids.

DIGESTIVE HEALTH: Herbal teas with benefits for

the digestive system include those containing ginger, peppermint, chamomile, and fennel. They can aid in the relief of bloating, gas, indigestion, nausea, and upset stomach symptoms. Probiotics, digestive enzymes, and apple cider vinegar are examples of natural treatments that can improve digestive health by balancing the gut flora, facilitating digestion, and easing gastrointestinal discomfort.

STRESS REDUCTION AND RELAXATION: Calming herbs such as passionflower, lemon balm, chamomile, and lavender can be added to herbal teas to help alleviate tension and encourage relaxation. Herbs that are known to help the body adapt to stress, such as rhodiola, holy basil, and ashwagandha, are examples of natural medicines that may promote emotional well-being.

SKIN CARE: Calendula, chamomile, lavender, and green tea, among other herbs, can be used in topical applications and beverages to nourish and soothe the skin, lower inflammation, and speed up the healing of wounds. Numerous skin disorders, including acne, eczema, and sunburn, can also be treated with natural medicines like coconut oil, shea butter, aloe vera gel, and witch hazel.

IMMUNE SUPPORT: To strengthen the immune system and lower the chance of infection, try taking herbal teas and supplements made with immune-supporting herbs like ginseng, echinacea, elderberry, and astragalus. Supplemental natural therapies like zinc, vitamin C, and medicinal mushrooms (like shiitake and reishi) may also strengthen immune system performance and increase defense against infections.

ENHANCEMENT OF SLEEP: Herbal teas with relaxing properties, such as lavender, chamomile, passionflower, and valerian, are frequently used to enhance the quality of sleep. Supplements, including melatonin, magnesium, and 5-HTP (5-hydroxytryptophan), are examples of natural therapies that may promote sound sleep patterns and help treat insomnia.

WEIGHT MANAGEMENT: Herbal teas with ingredients that speed up metabolism, such as dandelion root, green tea, and oolong tea, may aid in weight loss and metabolic control. When paired with a good diet and regular exercise, natural remedies like forskolin, conjugated linoleic acid (CLA), and chromium picolinate may help promote healthy weight management.

PAIN RELIEF: Herbal teas made with anti-inflammatory herbs like peppermint, ginger, and turmeric can help reduce pain brought on by ailments like arthritis, headaches, and tense muscles. For both acute and chronic pain, natural therapies including arnica, capsaicin, and CBD (cannabidiol) may be helpful.

RESPIRATORY HEALTH: Expectorant and decongestant herbal teas, such as those made with marshmallow root, thyme, licorice, and eucalyptus, can help ease the symptoms of colds, coughing, and respiratory congestion. Saline nasal irrigation and steam inhalation with essential oils (e.g., peppermint, eucalyptus) are examples of natural therapies that can help maintain respiratory health and unclog nasal passages.

HORMONAL BALANCE: Menstrual cycle regulation, PMS symptoms relief, and hormonal health may all be supported by herbal teas that contain hormone-balancing herbs such as black cohosh, red clover, chasteberry (Vitex), and dong quai. Maca root, evening primrose oil, and DIM (diindolylmethane) are examples of natural therapies that may be used to balance hormones and treat associated symptoms.

These are only a few of the numerous applications and

advantages of natural remedies and herbal drinks. While many people find success with these cures, it's important to remember that not everyone will benefit from them. It's also advisable to speak with a healthcare provider if you have any underlying medical concerns or are pregnant or nursing.

Incorporating Herbal Teas and Remedies into Daily Life

Incorporating herbal teas and treatments into daily life can be a fun way to improve general health and well-being. Here are a few methods for incorporating them:

HERBAL TEAS

- For a calming cup of tea to help you relax or get going in the morning, try chamomile or peppermint, or try ginger for a zingy start.

- To add flavor to grains like rice or quinoa, use herbal teas as a basis for cooking.

- In the warmer months, make cool herbal iced teas with blends like lemongrass or hibiscus.

COOKING AND CULINARY USES

- For extra flavor and health benefits, add fresh herbs to your dishes, such as rosemary, thyme, or basil.

- To season food, add dried herbs like parsley, sage, or oregano.

- Try preparing vinegars or oils infused with herbs to pour over roasted vegetables or salads.

AROMATHERAPY

- To create a relaxing or energizing ambiance at home, diffuse essential oils such as lavender, eucalyptus, or lemon.

- To relieve sinus congestion or encourage relaxation, add a few drops of essential oils to a bowl of hot water, then breathe in the steam.

- Make your own linen sprays or room sprays by diluting essential oils with water.

TOPICAL APPLICATIONS

- Calendula, comfrey, and lavender are good herbs to use in homemade herbal salves or balms to relieve mild skin irritations.

- To make massage oils for relaxation or muscle treatment, infuse herbs into carrier oils such as coconut or jojoba.

- Make potent herbal teas to serve as a foundation for DIY hair rinses and face toners.

TINCTURES AND SUPPLEMENTS

- For their health-promoting qualities, include ginseng, ashwagandha, or turmeric in your daily routine as herbal supplements.

- For convenient dosage, steep herbs in glycerin or alcohol for several weeks, filter, and store in dropper bottles to create your own herbal tinctures.

- For an additional nutritional boost, use liquid herbal extracts in juices, smoothies, or teas.

Always conduct an extensive study or speak with a medical practitioner before utilizing herbal treatments, particularly if you are expecting or breastfeeding a child, have any underlying medical concerns, or both.

Chapter Five

12 Herbal Teas Recipes

Here are 12 herbal tea recipes using various herbs, spices, and flavor combinations.

Refreshing Ginger Mint Tea

Ingredients:

1 tablespoon dried peppermint leaves

1 teaspoon dried ginger root slices

Honey for sweetness (optional)

Instructions:

- For 5-7 minutes, steep the dried ginger slices and peppermint leaves in hot water.

- If desired, strain and add honey or lemon.

- For a midday pick-me-up, sip on a refreshing cup of mint ginger tea.

Energizing Citrus Green Tea

Ingredients:

1 green tea bag or 1 teaspoon of loose green tea leaves

1 teaspoon of dried orange peel1 teaspoon dried lemon peel

Honey for sweetness (optional)

Instructions:

- For 3-5 minutes, steep the dried citrus peels and green tea in boiling water.

- If desired, strain and add honey for sweetness.

- Savor a refreshing cup of citrus green tea to start your day.

Rooibos Chai with Spices

Ingredients:

1 rooibos tea bag or 1 teaspoon loose rooibos tea leaves

1 cinnamon stick

3-4 whole cloves

2-3 cardamom pods

1 slice of fresh ginger

For a chai latte, milk and honey are optional.

Instructions:

- For 5-7 minutes, steep the Rooibos tea and spices in boiling water.

- If you would like a creamy chai latte, strain and add milk and honey.

- Warm yourself up with a cup of spiced rooibos tea on a cold afternoon.

Hibiscus Flower Rose Tea

Ingredients:

1 hibiscus tea bag or 1 teaspoon dried hibiscus flowers

1 teaspoon dried rose petals

1 teaspoon of dried chamomile flowers

Honey for sweetness (optional)

Instructions:

- For 5-7 minutes, steep the dried rose petals, chamomile flowers, and hibiscus tea in boiling water.

- Strain and sweeten with honey, if desired.

- Enjoy a fragrant cup of hibiscus flower rose tea as a calming evening beverage.

Nutritious Nettle Leaf Tea

Ingredients:

1 tablespoon dried nettle leaves

1 teaspoon dried lemon balm leaves

1 teaspoon dried mint leaves

Honey for sweetness (optional)

Instructions:

- For 5-7 minutes, steep the leaves of nettle, lemon balm, and mint in hot water.

- If desired, strain and add honey for sweetness.

- Savor a nutritious cup of nettle leaf tea for potential health benefits.

Calming Passionflower Tea with Lemon Balm

Ingredients:

1 tablespoon dried lemon balm leaves

1 teaspoon dried passionflower

Honey for sweetness (optional)

Instructions:

- For 5-7 minutes, steep the passionflower and lemon balm leaves in hot water.

- Strain and sweeten with honey, if desired.

- Before going to bed, have a soothing cup of lemon balm passionflower tea.

Immune-Supporting Echinacea Elderberry Tea

Ingredients:

1 echinacea tea bag or 1 teaspoon dried echinacea root

1 teaspoon dried elderberries

Honey and lemon for flavor (optional)

Instructions:

- For 5-7 minutes, steep the dried elderberries and echinacea tea in hot water.

- After straining, if preferred, add honey and lemon for flavor.

- In order to strengthen your immune system, sip on a nutritious cup of elderberry echinacea tea.

Digestive Herbal Tea

Ingredients:

1 tablespoon dried peppermint leaves

1 teaspoon dried fennel seeds

1 teaspoon dried ginger root slices

Honey for sweetness (optional)

Instructions:

- For 5-7 minutes, steep the dried ginger slices, fennel seeds, and peppermint leaves in hot water.

- If desired, strain and add honey for sweetness.

- After dinner, sip a comforting cup of herbal tea for digestion.

Refreshing Hibiscus Peppermint Tea

Ingredients:

1 hibiscus tea bag or 1 teaspoon dried hibiscus flowers

1 tablespoon dried peppermint leaves

Honey for sweetness (optional)

Instructions:

- For 5-7 minutes, steep the dried peppermint leaves and hibiscus tea in hot water.

- If desired, strain and add honey for sweetness.

- Savor the refreshing and moisturizing qualities of hibiscus peppermint tea with delight.

Refreshing Cucumber Mint Tea

Ingredients:

1 green tea bag or 1 teaspoon of loose green tea leaves

3-4 slices of fresh cucumber

2-3 fresh mint leaves

Honey for sweetness (optional)

Instructions:

- For 3–5 minutes, steep the green tea, cucumber slices, and fresh mint leaves in hot water.

- If desired, strain and add honey for sweetness.

- On a hot summer's day, sip a refreshing cup of cucumber mint tea.

Calming Chamomile Lavender Tea

Ingredients:

1 tablespoon dried chamomile flowers

1 teaspoon dried lavender buds

1 teaspoon dried lemon balm leaves

1 teaspoon dried peppermint leaves

Instructions:

- Give the herbs a 5-7 minute steep in hot water.

- Before going to bed, strain and savor a calming cup of chamomile lavender tea.

Anti-inflammatory Turmeric Ginger Tea

Ingredients:

1 teaspoon turmeric powder or grated fresh turmeric root

1 teaspoon grated fresh ginger

1 teaspoon of honey

1 teaspoon of lemon juice

A pinch of black pepper (to improve the absorption of turmeric)

Coconut milk for creaminess (optional)

Instructions:

- For 5-7 minutes, steep the turmeric and grated ginger in hot water.

- After straining, mix in the lemon juice, honey, and black pepper.

- Coconut milk can be used, if desired, for a creamy

texture.

- Warm up with a cup of anti-inflammatory turmeric and ginger tea.

Feel free to change the component proportions and flavorings to your liking. These herbal tea recipes have a wide range of flavors and potential health benefits, making them ideal for sipping and savoring throughout the day. Enjoy discovering the world of herbal teas!

10 Natural Remedies Recipes

Here are ten recipes for natural remedies that you can try.

Ginger Lemon Honey Tea

Ingredients: fresh ginger, lemon slices, and honey.

Instructions:

- Cut ginger into slices and boil in water.

- Pour into a cup after straining.

- To taste, add honey and lemon slices.

- Savor it, warm or cold.

Calendula Balm

Ingredients: dried calendula flowers, coconut oil, and beeswax;

Instructions:

- Use a double boiler to infuse the dried calendula flowers in the coconut oil.

- Filter and combine with liquefied beeswax.

- Transfer to containers and allow to solidify.

- As needed, apply it to minor skin irritations.

Turmeric Milky Mix

Ingredients: milk (plant-based or dairy), honey, cinnamon, and black pepper

Instructions:

- In a saucepan, heat the milk and then add the cinnamon, turmeric, and a dash of black pepper.

- Use honey to sweeten.

- Mix well and savor prior to going to bed.

Peppermint Oil Steam Inhalation

Ingredients: peppermint essential oil, hot water

Instructions:

- Pour some hot water into a dish and add a few drops of peppermint oil.

- To release congestion, lean over the bowl, cover

your head with a towel, and breathe in the steam.

Elderberry Syrup

Ingredients: dried elderberries, water, honey, cinnamon, and cloves

Instructions:

- Simmer dried elderberries with water, cinnamon, and cloves until reduced by half.

- Filter and combine with honey.

- Take one tablespoon daily for immune support and store it in the refrigerator.

Chamomile Lavender Relaxation Bath Soak

Ingredients: Epsom salt, dried lavender buds, and dried chamomile flowers.

Instructions:

- Combine equal amounts of Epsom salt, dried lavender buds, and dried chamomile flowers.

- Add it to a warm bath and soak for relaxation and stress relief.

Arnica Massage Oil

Ingredients: carrier oil (almond or jojoba oil), arnica flowers

Instructions:

- Use a double boiler to infuse dried arnica flowers into carrier oil.

- Strain and apply as a massage oil to relieve aching joints and muscles.

Thyme Cough Syrup

Ingredients: fresh thyme sprigs, honey

Instructions:

- Simmer fresh thyme sprigs in water until reduced by half. Filter and mix with honey.

- Take a teaspoon as needed to relieve sore throats and coughs.

Lemon Balm Lip Moisturizer

Ingredients: beeswax, coconut oil, and dried lemon balm leaves.

Instructions:

- Use a double boiler to infuse dried lemon balm leaves into coconut oil.

- Filter and combine with liquefied beeswax.

- Transfer it into moisturizer containers and allow it to harden.

Nettle Leaf Hair Wash

Ingredients: water, apple cider vinegar, and dried nettle leaves

Instructions:

- Soak dried nettle leaves for a few weeks in a solution of apple cider vinegar and water.

- To encourage healthy hair development and scalp health, strain it and use it as a hair wash.

Prior to widespread application, it is advisable to conduct a patch test on a small area of skin, particularly if you have sensitive skin or allergies. In the event of any negative side effects, cease usage immediately.

ACKNOWLEDGEMENTS

All glory belongs to God. I'd also want to thank my wonderful family, partner, fans, readers, friends, and customers for their constant support and words of encouragement.

www.ingramcontent.com/pod-product-compliance
Lightning Source LLC
Chambersburg PA
CBHW031134020426
42333CB00012B/367